Newcastle
City Council

Health and
Wellbeing

Newcastle Libraries and Information Service

☎ **0845 002 0336**

Due for return	Due for return	Due for return

Please return this item to any of Newcastle's Libraries by the last
date shown above. ff not requested by another customer the loan
can be renewed, you can do this by phone, post or in person.
Charges may be made for late returns.

THIS IS A CARLTON BOOK

Text and design copyright © 2008
Carlton Books Limited

This edition published by
Carlton Books Limited 2008
20 Mortimer Street
London W1T 3JW

ISBN 978-1-84732-226-5

Printed and bound in Singapore

Senior Executive Editor: Lisa Dyer
Senior Art Editor: Gulen Shevki-Taylor
Designer: Zoë Dissell
Production: Kate Pimm

Your **Carbon Footprint** is the amount of carbon dioxide emitted
due to your daily activities – from washing a load of laundry to
driving to work. See www.carbonfootprint.com for ways to reduce
your impact on the environment.

the
little
GREEN
BOOK
of

Health

SARAH CALLARD

250
TIPS
FOR AN
ECO
LIFESTYLE

CARLTON
BOOKS

Leading a healthy life and living an eco-friendly lifestyle often go hand in hand – what's better for you is usually best for the planet, too. This book is full of suggestions on how to improve your health by avoiding exposure to toxins and chemicals in the world around you. It also explores healthy living ideas that won't cost the planet and the benefits of using natural remedies for minor ailments.

1 ON YOUR BIKE

Leave the car behind and get on your bike. A 30-minute commute by bike will burn 8 calories a minute or 11 kg (24 lb) of fat a year, according to the international non-profit Friends of the Earth. You will also be helping the environment because you will save around 1 kg (2 lb) of carbon dioxide for every 8 km (5 m) trip taken by bike rather than car.

2 LEAD A LESS SEDENTARY LIFE

By getting out into the countryside you will be improving your health and wellbeing, and as long as you use public transport, cycle or walk, you will not be harming the environment. Research has found that the more time we spend in nature the more likely we are to try and protect it.

3 GO FOR A WALK

Improve your health and boost your fitness by going for a walk, every day if possible. Research has shown that regular walking is associated with reduced mortality for older and younger adults, as well as a reduction in the risk of cardiovascular disease and bone strength.

4 MIND HOW YOU GO

Walk your next journey rather than hopping in the car. Walking has been shown to improve mental health by boosting self-esteem, relieving symptoms of depression and anxiety, and offering opportunities for relaxation and social contact. It is also environmentally friendly.

5 AVOID THE GYM

Unless you live next door, avoid the gym. Instead, improve your health and fitness by walking or running. Gyms have a significant impact on the environment due to the energy they use for lighting, air conditioning and heating. There is also the added environmental impact of people driving to the gym and home again.

6 SCRAP THE SCHOOL RUN

For the sake of your and your children's health, and the impact on the environment, try a different approach to the school run. If you can, why not walk or use public transport? If none of these are practical, pool resources with other parents and take it in turns to drop off and pick up the children to cut back on multiple car journeys.

7

TURN OFF THE COMPUTER

Research has found that only half of 11 to 16 year olds currently walk for ten minutes in a day. Children walk significantly less than they did 50 years ago and there are considerably more overweight and obese children. Encourage them to switch off and get out – it will save energy and improve their health.

8

GET ACTIVE EARLY

One of the best things you can do to improve your children's health and the environment is to get them active early on. If children experience walking as part of a fun activity, they will want to do it again. Aim for something that will appeal to them, such as a few hours at a playground or boating pond.

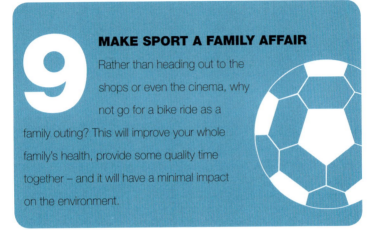

9 MAKE SPORT A FAMILY AFFAIR

Rather than heading out to the shops or even the cinema, why not go for a bike ride as a family outing? This will improve your whole family's health, provide some quality time together – and it will have a minimal impact on the environment.

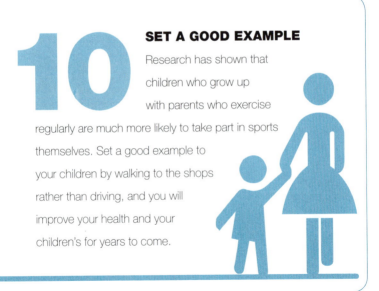

10 SET A GOOD EXAMPLE

Research has shown that children who grow up with parents who exercise regularly are much more likely to take part in sports themselves. Set a good example to your children by walking to the shops rather than driving, and you will improve your health and your children's for years to come.

11 LEAVE THE CAR FOR SHORT JOURNEYS

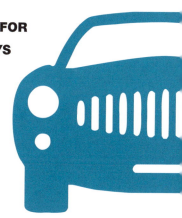

Nearly 40% of journeys of less than 3 km (2 m) are made by car, even though these are the kinds of distances that could be cycled quite easily. Short car trips result in higher levels of emissions because engines are not operating at their optimum temperature.

12 JOIN A CONSERVATION GROUP

A good way to help improve the environment and your health is to join a local conservation group. This will ensure that you spend time outside helping to maintain the environment at the same time as improving your health and general wellbeing.

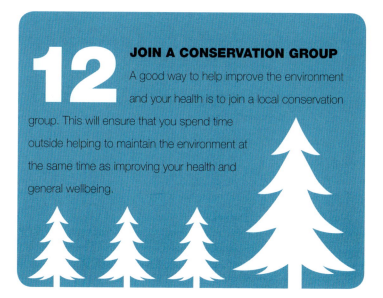

13 CYCLE TO SCHOOL

Get your children on their bikes and cycling to school. This will help improve their health as well as reduce carbon emissions. Make sure they take part in a cycling course first to ensure that they are proficient and confident on the roads.

14 JOIN A GREEN GYM

The Green Gym project is a scheme to encourage people to get fit at the same time as improving the environment. It offers 3-hour sessions of physical activity in the outdoors. There are Green Gym groups in the UK, Australia and the US, and there is always scope to set one up yourself locally.

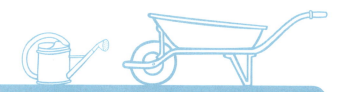

15 GARDEN AWAY STRESS

Research has shown that gardening is a great way to relieve stress and may help combat depression. There are even claims that a harmless bacteria normally found in dirt, *Mycobacterium vaccae,* has been found to boost the production of serotonin, a mood-regulating brain chemical.

16 GET AN ALLOTMENT

Growing your own vegetables will be better for your health and the environment. You will reduce your carbon footprint by avoiding car journeys to the supermarkets and can ensure that the food you eat is free from pesticides and other chemicals.

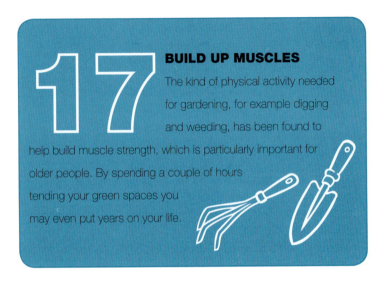

17

BUILD UP MUSCLES

The kind of physical activity needed for gardening, for example digging and weeding, has been found to help build muscle strength, which is particularly important for older people. By spending a couple of hours tending your green spaces you may even put years on your life.

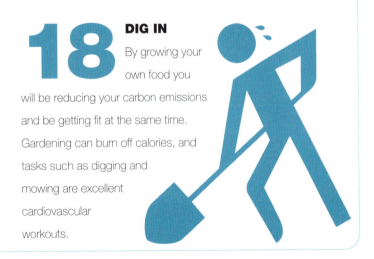

18

DIG IN

By growing your own food you will be reducing your carbon emissions and be getting fit at the same time. Gardening can burn off calories, and tasks such as digging and mowing are excellent cardiovascular workouts.

19

BURN GREEN CALORIES

Go green and burn off more calories by gardening than visiting the gym. Research has shown that almost a third more calories can be burnt in an hour of gardening than would be done in a step aerobics class. Other household tasks, such as washing dishes or painting the house, also burn calories effectively.

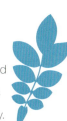

20

MAKE YOUR OWN COMPOST

Reduce waste and make your own compost for your garden. It takes around six months for food and garden waste to break down to form usable compost; however, the process can be helped along by turning the compost over regularly. This will provide regular exercise and help to improve your general fitness and muscle strength, too.

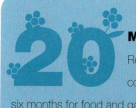

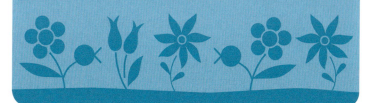

21

GET FIT WITH PHYTOESTROGENS

Plant phytoestrogens are natural hormone balancers and they may improve hormonal health in women going through the menopause. Soya, legumes, seeds and lentils all contain phytoestrogens, which balance hormones naturally as well as offering protection against breast cancer and heart disease.

22

BALANCE HORMONES WITH BLACK COHOSH

The herb black cohosh was used by Native Americans as a traditional folk remedy for womens' health conditions, such as menstrual cramps and hot flashes, arthritis, muscle pain, sore throat and indigestion, and today is used by some women to help them through the menopause. It balances hormones without the health risks associated with HRT.

23 USE ORGANIC SANITARY PROTECTION

Avoid exposure to the chemicals used in conventional sanitary protection such as chlorine, which has been linked to toxic shock syndrome, and dioxins, which are known to be carcinogenic. Choose 100% organic and GM-free cotton products, such as those by Natracare, which will be kinder to you and the environment.

24 BIN THE WIPES

Feminine wipes are totally unnecessary and may even be damaging to your health. Save money, reduce waste and avoid exposure to potentially toxic chemicals such as fragrances and preservatives, which are often derived from petrochemicals, and go natural instead. If you must use them, seek out organic cotton wipes.

25 EASE PERIOD PAIN WITH YOGA

Gentle exercise helps the body get rid of excess hormones and flush them out of the body. Yoga in particular also helps to balance the endocrine system and has the added benefit of reducing stress and improving mood.

26 HELP HOT FLUSHES WITH SAGE

Research has shown that one of the main symptoms of the menopause, hot flushes, can be helped by supplementing with sage. This herb is a natural product that can be taken in tincture or capsule form and helps the body to rebalance the sweat-regulating mechanism in the brain naturally.

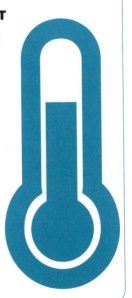

27 DON'T HAVE A MID-LIFE CRISIS

Approach the menopause naturally and avoid hormone replacement therapy (HRT) if possible Hormones from medicines have been detected in waterways and HRT has been linked to ovarian and breast cancer. Prepare yourself for a healthy menopause by eating a balanced diet and reducing stress.

28 A MAGNETIC FORCE

Avoid using unnecessary drugs for hormone problems by using a magnetic device known as Ladycare. A magnet that clips onto underwear over the abdomen, it has been found to reduce menopausal symptoms as well as PMS and other hormonal health problems.

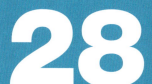

29 SCRUB UP

Detox naturally with a body brush. Use a wooden brush with natural bristles to give your body a good brush – this will improve circulation and aid detoxification, with very little impact on the environment.

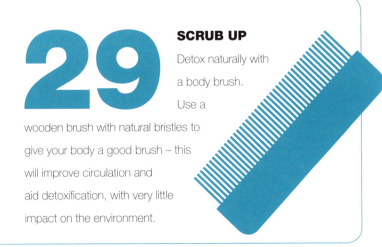

30 FIGHT NAUSEA WITH GINGER

Ginger is one of the best known natural remedies for nausea. It is particularly beneficial for morning sickness in early pregnancy. Pour boiling water over fresh ginger root to make a tea, and drink it first thing in the morning. Alternatively, nibble on stem ginger.

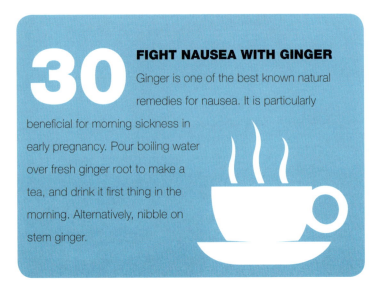

31

REDUCE BLOATING WITH GENTIAN

A digestive tonic, the plant *Gentiana lutea* contains one of the most bitter substances known, and bitters are used in herbalism to improve appetite and digestion. Gentian is believed to aid digestion by increasing salivary flow and easing bloating, and has the added benefit of strengthening the pancreas and spleen. If It can be taken as a tincture or brewed into an herbal tea.

32

BOOST DIGESTION WITH PROBIOTICS

If you have digestion problems such as bloating and flatulence, avoid over-the-counter medicines and treat the condition naturally with probiotics instead. Natural live yogurt is ideal for increasing the healthy bacteria in your system on a day-to-day basis and if you need a boost, for example after a course of antibiotics, try supplements as well.

33 NATURALLY ON THE MOVE

If you suffer from constipation, avoid traditional laxatives, which can sometimes exacerbate the problem, and get moving with natural laxatives such as psyllium husks. A tablespoon of these or ground flaxseeds sprinkled on cereal in the morning should ease the problem quickly.

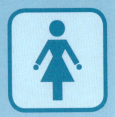

34 STOP SMOKING

If you haven't already, quit smoking. Research has shown that it takes ten years for a cigarette butt to decay. The health implications of smoking such as premature ageing are well known, as are the effects of passive smoking, so stop now for the sake of your health and the planet's.

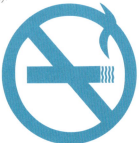

35

FRESHEN BREATH WITH ALOE VERA

Serious cases of bad breath, or halitosis, may be caused by stomach disorders. Daily gargling with aloe vera juice will help to reduce toxins in the digestive system as well as relieving any inflammation. Look out for an organic variety, however, to ensure it is toxin-free and kind to the environment.

36

CHEW PARSLEY

Instead of using harsh mouthwashes to freshen your breath, chew on some fresh parsley. Traditionally used to disguise the smell of alcohol on breath because of its natural breath-freshening properties, parsley contains high levels of chlorophyll, which helps prevent toxins from accumulating in the digestive tract.

37 CHOOSE A HOLISTIC DENTIST

Mercury in the amalgam used in traditional dental fillings has been associated with a wide range of health problems, including headaches and even depression. If possible, choose a holistic dentist who uses homeopathic techniques and avoids mercury amalgam fillings altogether. You could also consider getting your existing amalgam fillings replaced with a mercury-free white-composite alternative.

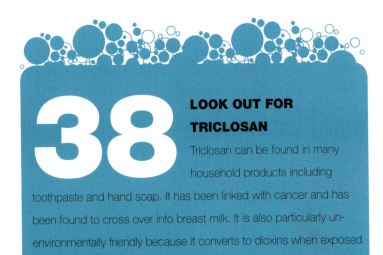

38 LOOK OUT FOR TRICLOSAN

Triclosan can be found in many household products including toothpaste and hand soap. It has been linked with cancer and has been found to cross over into breast milk. It is also particularly un-environmentally friendly because it converts to dioxins when exposed to sunlight and is known to be toxic to aquatic organisms.

39

AVOID SLS FOR BETTER HEALTH

Sodium laurel sulphate (SLS) is a common ingredient in many household products from shampoo to detergent, but it has been linked to a number of health concerns including cancer and is a known skin irritant. Avoid it by making sure you use plant-based products, which are also kinder to the environment.

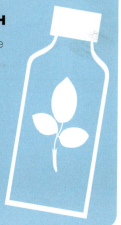

40

BEWARE PEGS

Look out for ingredients called polyethylene glycol (known as PEGs) in bodycare products. Polyethylene glycol is a commercial polyether used in many skin creams, toothpastes and sexual lubricants. Studies have highlighted that some PEGs may cause dermatitis and other skin irritations, while research has found that a carcinogen may be formed as a by-product during manufacture.

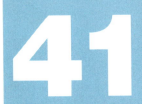

41

HAVE SAFE, GREEN SEX

Use a biodegradable condom from the manufacturer Condomi. Condoms pose a waste problem and, when they are not disposed of properly, they end up polluting our public places and marine environments. So choose green and ethical condoms – they are also vegan – for safer, eco-friendly sex.

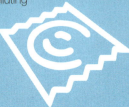

AVOID HARSH PET SHAMPOOS

Research has found a link between pet shampoos that contain a type of harsh detergent called pyrethrins to autism in children. The research, published in the *New Scientist*, found that mothers of children with autism-spectrum disorder were twice as likely to have reported using pet shampoos as those of healthy children.

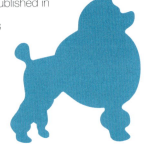

43 MAKE YOUR OWN TOILETRIES

Avoid exposure to toiletries containing harsh detergents, which can cause skin sensitivity and other health problems, and make your own. Store-cupboard staples such as honey and olive oil can be mixed with an egg yolk to create a homemade conditioner; and try avocado mashed with natural yogurt for a facemask.

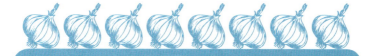

44 TREAT DANDRUFF NATURALLY

Anti-dandruff shampoos contain a cocktail of chemicals, so avoid these and make your own herbal remedy. Simmer some garlic, nettles and thyme in a pot for five minutes, then cool and strain. Use the mixture as a final rinse every time you wash your hair.

45 BOOST HEALTH WITH MEDITATION

Research has shown that regular meditation is thought to have a broad range of benefits for the mind and body: it boosts the immune system, improves sleep, and is beneficial for insomnia, obesity and depression.

46 CUT CAFFEINE FOR BETTER IMMUNITY

For a healthy immune system, avoid caffeine and alcohol. Coffee, tea and colas are stimulants and known to compromise the immune system, making you more susceptible to viruses, coughs and colds. Caffeine increases the heart rate and elevates blood pressure, plus stimulates the excretion of the stress hormones cortisol, epinephrine and norepinephrine. Drink health-promoting herbal teas instead.

47 SOOTHE CYSTITIS WITH CRANBERRIES

Drinking cranberry juice is a natural way to prevent and ease the pain of cystitis without having to resort to antibiotics. Research has found that as much as 80% of all the bacteria in the body is resistant to conventional treatment – generally antibiotics – which may also cause other problems such as thrush. It is thought that the cranberry juice works by preventing bacteria from adhering to the walls of the bladder, and so preventing infection taking hold.

48 CURE THRUSH WITH YOGURT

Natural, live yogurt is good for lots of minor health problems, including thrush. The yogurt contains *Lactobacillus acidophilus* which, like yeasts, naturally live in the human body, and its presence helps keep Candida yeast populations in check. It can be eaten or applied topically to the affected area. Tea tree oil added to the bath can also help get rid of fungal infections.

49

EASE ECZEMA WITH SUPPLEMENTS

Research has found that low levels of zinc and calcium may be linked to an increased risk of eczema so boost levels naturally by increasing your intake of organic leafy greens and supplementing with zinc or calcium tablets.

50

EFAS FOR ECZEMA

Research has found that essential fatty acids (EFAs) may play a significant role in keeping skin healthy and may help to ease the symptoms associated with eczema and psoriasis. Boost levels of essential fatty acids by increasing the amount of fatty fish such as salmon or linseeds in your diet.

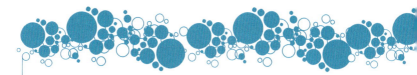

51 AVOID OVEN CLEANERS

Conventional oven cleaners often contain a number of highly toxic chemicals including sodium hydroxide, and contact with these chemicals could cause serious damage to your health. To avoid any risk, use a homemade combination of salt and bicarbonate of soda (baking soda) mixed with a little lemon juice or vinegar.

52 KEEP YOUR BULBS DUST FREE

Dust in the home can trigger allergies and lead to respiratory problems. Make sure you keep your light fittings dust-free, as this will create a healthier environment and it will also make each bulb more efficient, thereby saving energy.

53

BOOST IMMUNITY
WITH ASTRAGALUS

Although less well known than echinacea, the Chinese herb astragalus is very beneficial for boosting immune health. Traditionally used in Chinese herbal medicine, it is thought to stimulate white blood cell production, which supports the immune system by fighting infections.

54

BEAT EXAM STRESS
WITH RHODIOLA

The herb rhodiola (*Rhodiola rosea*) has been found to improve mental health naturally. It is an adaptogenic herb, which means it helps the body cope with stress and a demanding lifestyle. This makes it ideal for exam times, the menopause or simply busy periods in your life.

55

GET AHEAD

Boost concentration and ease headaches and eyestrain with an Indian head massage. This is a traditional technique designed to invigorate and stimulate the senses as well as to relax and heal aches and pains. Because it is thought to help boost concentration levels and sharpen the mind, it is an ideal pre-exam or pr-interview therapy.

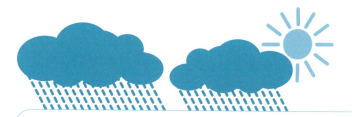

56

TREAT DEPRESSION NATURALLY

Antidepressants do have some side effects and there are concerns about them being overprescribed. Research has found that the herb St John's Wort (*Hypericum perforatum*) is as effective at relieving mild to moderate depression as antidepressants, but without the side effects.

57 PACK IN THE PANIC ATTACKS

If you suffer from panic attacks and anxiety, you may like to try the natural dietary supplement 5-HTP (hydroxytryptophan). Found in minute amounts in such foods as turkey and cheese, 5-HTP is an amino acid and works by increasing the serotonin in the brain in a similar way to antidepressants and beta-blockers, but without the side effects. It may also be beneficial as an appetite suppressant and sleep aid.

58 GREENER CLEANERS

Reducing your reliance on chemical cleaners can improve your health as well as the environment. Research has found that only around 14% of the most heavily used chemicals have basic safety data publicly available, so it's difficult to know exactly what you and your family are coming into contact with.

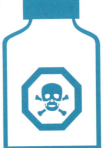

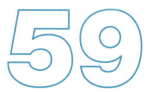

FORMALDEHYDE WARNING

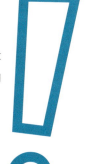

This is a common ingredient in lots of different household and body-care products. It is a suspected human carcinogen and has been found to cause lung cancer in rats. It has also been linked to asthma and headaches. Formaldehyde is often found in disinfectants and is used as a preservative in deodorants and hand wash.

60

REACH FOR THE RHUBARB

Avoid using harsh detergents which have been linked to a number of health problems including asthma, and which are damaging to the environment. Instead, remove burnt-on food and grease from the bottom of pans by boiling up rhubarb stalks, which will do the job just as well.

61 CHAMOMILE FOR COLIC

Add some drops of chamomile essential oil to a warm bath to help ease a colicky baby. Chamomile is a gentle sedative and anti-spasmodic so will help to calm and soothe. If you prefer, add a couple of drops of oil to a carrier oil, such as almond oil, and massage your baby instead.

62 NATURAL TEETHERS

Instead of giving your baby plastic teethers why not try offering them pieces of frozen banana – it will disintegrate as they chew. Other natural teething aids include crusts of toast and strips of organic dried fruit such as mango.

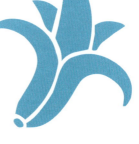

63

HOMEOPATHIC HELP

Homeopathy is really helpful for treating health problems in babies and young children because it is safe. For a teething baby use the remedy Chamomilla. Either dissolve a pill in water and give teaspoonful by teaspoonful until the symptoms subside, or alternatively use homeopathic teething granules, a product that mothers highly recommend.

64

CUT OUT THE CHEMICALS IF YOU ARE PREGNANT

Recent research found that children born to women who used lots of cleaning products and air fresheners during pregnancy were more likely to have symptoms such as wheezing. It may sound obvious, but try simply opening windows to freshen rooms rather than using air fresheners.

65

EASE TEETHING WITH AMBER

If your baby is teething, avoid plastic teething rings. Instead, try an amber teething necklace. These are designed to be worn, not chewed, and act as a natural analgesic, easing the pain of teething when worn on the skin. However, babies must be supervised at all times while wearing the necklace.

66

GIVE BABIES A BREAK

Don't sterilize baby equipment using chemicals. Babies need to be able to develop their immune systems, so washing equipment with hot, soapy water and then rinsing with boiling water is sufficient. This simple method also reduces the amount of chemicals entering the waterways.

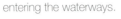

67

POLYCARBONATE WARNING

There are concerns about plastic baby feeding bottles made with polycarbonate plastic. A report in 2000 by the World Wildlife Fund highlighted the dangers posed by bisphenol-A (BPA), a hormone-disrupting chemical contained in polycarbonate that is particularly risky for children. Polycarbonate can be identified by looking on the packaging for PC7, or inside the recycling triangle for the number 7.

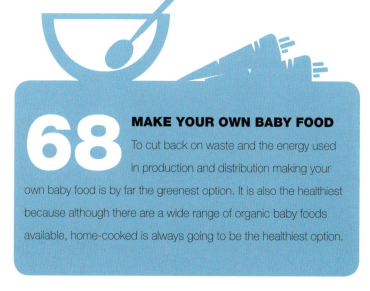

68

MAKE YOUR OWN BABY FOOD

To cut back on waste and the energy used in production and distribution making your own baby food is by far the greenest option. It is also the healthiest because although there are a wide range of organic baby foods available, home-cooked is always going to be the healthiest option.

69

USE WASHABLE NAPPIES

Protect your baby's health by ensuring that they don't come into contact with any chemicals from disposable nappies (diapers). Washable nappies help reduce the number of chemicals your baby is exposed to and they are better for the environment.

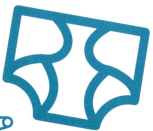

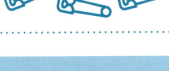

70

AVOID HARSH DETERGENTS

If you use washable nappies, avoid cleaning them with harsh detergents, which have been to linked to an increased sensitivity among some children. Choose a natural detergent, which is free from dyes and fragrances and is made from plant-based ingredients.

71 CHOOSE TO BREASTFEED

If you are having a baby, choose to breastfeed if you are able. Breastfeeding offers a significant number of major health benefits for you and baby. Environmentally, it's better too, because it requires no sterilizing solutions or equipment, and no plastic bottles, teats or containers.

72 DRESS YOUR BABY IN ORGANIC WOOL

Organic merino wool is non-allergenic, so as well as being kinder to the environment (and the sheep), it is also better for your little one. The wool helps regulate body temperature, enabling your baby to maintain a safe temperature, whether the weather is hot or cold.

73 HOMEOPATHY FOR KIDS

Avoid exposing your children to unnecessary medicines. Instead of reaching for painkillers such as Calpol or Tylenol, try homeopathy instead. It can be very effective for teething and colic pain, which are common reasons for administering painkillers for children, and it is safe enough to be used on babies.

74 USE A TALC ALTERNATIVE

Research suggests that using talcum powder may increase your risk of developing cancer. Look for natural alternatives or make your own using cornstarch mixed with a few drops of essential oils, particularly if you are considering using it on an infant or child.

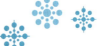

75 SOOTHE SKIN WITH CALENDULA

The herb calendula has antiviral properties and is good for soothing irritated skin. Calendula cream is ideal for use on babies with nappy (diaper) rash. Alternatively, make a soothing tea by pouring hot water over dried calendula and use the strained liquid to dab on minor skin infections.

76 TAKE UP SPORT AS A HOBBY

The best way to improve your health is to incorporate some regular exercise into your lifestyle. Taking up a sport as a hobby can help improve your fitness without any negative impact on the environment. Look out for local swimming, yoga or Pilates classes that you can walk to.

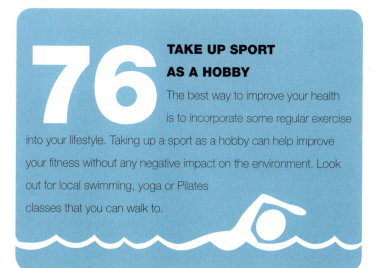

77

TAKE ADVANTAGE OF LOCAL AMENITIES

Rather than driving somewhere for a walk or a day out, take advantage of your local sports facilities, such as tennis courts. As long as you can walk or cycle to your local tennis court or swimming pool this is a very eco-friendly way to improve your health.

78

PLAN A HEALTHY AND GREEN HOLIDAY

Decline the two-week package to the islands and make your holiday healthy and green. Pack up your camping equipment and explore the coastline by bike or foot (with the help of public transport for longer distances). Children love camping and it's a very low-impact way to take a vacation.

79

CHOOSE A LOW-IMPACT ACTIVITY HOLIDAY

Why not combine getting healthy with taking your summer break? Rather than sitting back and having it all done for you, get active. Canal boat trips, hiking excursions and surfing vacations will be fun and improve your health and fitness at the same time.

80

CHOOSE AN ECO-FRIENDLY SPORT

There are plenty of sports and activities that will improve your health and boost your appreciation of the environment without having a negative impact on it. Surfing, climbing, walking and cycling are all about being outside and in harmony with the environment.

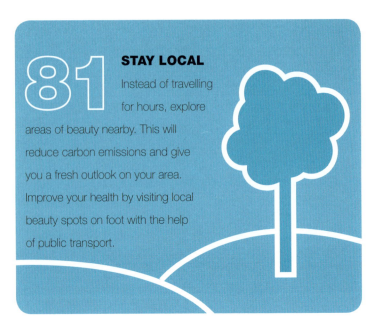

81 STAY LOCAL

Instead of travelling for hours, explore areas of beauty nearby. This will reduce carbon emissions and give you a fresh outlook on your area. Improve your health by visiting local beauty spots on foot with the help of public transport.

82 BECOME A RAMBLER

Spend your spare time rambling – regular brisk walking can improve your heart rate and circulation as well as lower blood pressure and reduce cholesterol levels. Some research has found that it can dramatically reduce the risk of heart attack.

83 GET A DOG

Having to walk a dog is one of the best ways to ensure that you get out and about in the countryside. A daily walk is extremely beneficial for your health, improving cardiovascular fitness; as long as you don't drive the dog to its walking spot, it's eco-friendly, too.

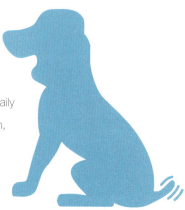

84 AVOID AIR TRAVEL

Air travel is one of the biggest contributors to global warming – in the UK it accounts for more than 6% of total carbon emissions. New research has also found that flying could be bad for the health due to contaminated air being pumped around the aircraft. The air absorbs fumes from the engine oil, and can cause nausea and headaches.

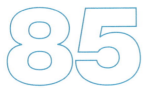

WIND DOWN
YOUR WINDOW

Air conditioning has been linked with a number of minor health problems. Avoid switching it on in your car when you are travelling at lower speeds. Tests have shown that it is more environmentally friendly to open your windows under speeds of 96 kph (60 mph) than it is to use air conditioning, which boosts fuel consumption.

TAKE A GREENER COMMUTE

If you are one of the many people who travel to work in a car on your own – the majority of work commutes are done by car – then leave it at home for a couple of days of the week.

Walking or cycling to work, or to the train station for longer journeys, will boost your cardiovascular health and help the environment.

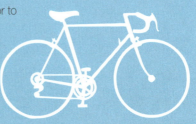

87 GET OUT AT LUNCHTIME

A staggering number of workers spend their lunch hour in the same position as the rest of their day – eating in front of their computers. If this applies to you, try switching off and going for a walk instead. A ten-minute walk will boost circulation and has been found to improve brain power, too.

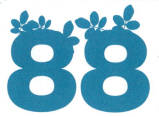

88 PUT A PLANT ON YOUR DESK

Research has shown that having a plant on your desk at work can help reduce your risk of getting a sore throat and stuffed-up nose. A study by researchers in Norway found that nose, throat and dry skin symptoms were 23% lower in offices with greenery.

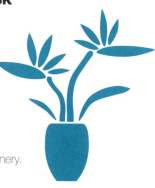

89

MOVE YOUR DESK TO THE WINDOW

Reduce your reliance on artificial lighting and cut carbon emissions by making the most of natural light. Place your desk by the window – research from Sweden has shown that sitting by the window is good for improving the mood, too.

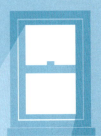

90

REDUCE YOUR USE OF THE PRINTER

Only switch on your printer when you need it. New research has found that printers can cause a form of indoor air pollution because they release tiny particles of toner-like material into the air, which could be inhaled into the lungs.

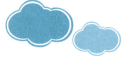

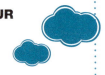

91

HAZARDS IN THE WORKPLACE

You may be aware of the environmental risks to your health in your own home, but what about your workplace? Many employees are exposed to waste materials and toxins without being fully aware. Check your company's health and safety guidelines, as well as your national standard; for example, the Occupational Safety and Health Administration (www.osha.gov) in the USA or try the Health and Safety Executive (www.hse.gov.uk) in the UK.

USE A CERAMIC MUG FOR YOUR TEA

Avoid using polystyrene cups for hot drinks when you are out and about. The waste problem they pose is considerable, especially when you consider that polystyrene cups never biodegrade. Also, there is some evidence that chemicals from the polystyrene may leach into the contents.

93 STRIKE OUT ON YOUR OWN

Consider going freelance! It's a lot easier to be green if you are working alone from home rather than in an office – there's no carbon emissions caused by the commute for a start. Research has shown that self-employed people report higher levels of job satisfaction and less stress.

94 TURN YOUR OFFICE GREEN, LITERALLY!

Studies have shown that offices painted white, blue or green are conducive to better mood and job satisfaction than other colours, particularly red. Just make sure you use a plant-based, low-VOC (volotile organic compound) paint.

95 USE THE STAIRS

Instead of using the lift (elevator) at work, walk up the stairs. This will cut energy use and improve your health instantly. Studies have shown that people who use the stairs have lower cholesterol, better breathing capacity, healthier hearts and weigh less.

96 TAKE A BREAK

Save energy by switching your computer off and taking regular breaks throughout the day. We waste a huge amount of energy by leaving appliances on standby, so turn your computer off and have a rest. Long periods in front of the machine can lead to carpal tunnel syndrome and even deep-vein thrombosis.

97 RESTRICT YOUR USE OF LAPTOPS

Although laptops use up to 80% less energy than desktop computers, they may be responsible for more health problems. There is evidence that they can cause injuries from bad posture and they have also been linked to fertility problems. So if you have a laptop, try not to use it for extended periods on your lap.

98 SCRAP THE AIR CON

Lobby your boss to eschew energy-guzzling air conditioning for more simple methods, such as installing blinds and opening the windows. Air conditioning has been linked with minor ailments such as colds and coughs; it also means you have to adjust to the temperature outside every time you leave your office.

99 EASE STRESS WITH SOUND THERAPY

Sound therapy works by using brass or crystal bowls to produce sounds that are thought to aid relaxation. It is believed to benefit a number of health problems including stress, insomnia, depression and even irritable bowel syndrome.

100 TREAT BACK PAIN WITH THE BOWEN TECHNIQUE

The Bowen technique is a holistic therapy that is reportedly most successful for treating problems such as back pain, frozen shoulders and neck pain – all which can be brought on by long hours in front of a computer. It is also thought to be beneficial for hay fever, asthma and migraines. The therapist uses fingers or thumbs to manipulate muscles with a gentle rolling motion.

101

TURN ON YOUR HEAD

Relieve aches and pains with inversion therapy. It may sound odd, but hanging upside-down can relieve a aches and pains, stiffness and stress. It is also thought to help the body detox by speeding up the flow of blood and lymphatic fluids that clear out waste.

102

LOWER BLOOD PRESSURE WITH TAI CHI

Studies have found that the traditional Chinese practise of tai chi can help to reduce blood pressure in women. It was also found to improve balance, reduce anxiety and stress, and improve flexibility. It is considered to be a particularly beneficial exercise for middle-aged adults.

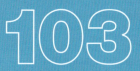

103 DRINK MORE WATER

Most of us could do with drinking more water. Being dehydrated adversely affects your mental performance. When dehydrated, your attention and concentration decrease by 13% and short-term memory by 7%. Make sure you drink filtered tap water rather than bottled to reduce bottle waste.

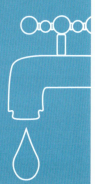

104 HAVE A CUP OF ORGANIC TEA

Research has found that the antioxidants in regular black tea can help to improve heart health and may even protect against cancer. Tea is a natural product but choose an organic variety to help protect the environment against over-use of pesticides and fertilizers.

105 SPICE IT UP

Research has found that cayenne pepper and turmeric can be beneficial for pain relief from joint and muscle strain. Topical creams containing cayenne are best for sore muscles but it can also be taken in tincture form for fast-acting relief, and it can be included as a spice in food. Turmeric can be used as a spice in food or taken in a capsule form.

106 TAKE THE STING OUT OF ARTHRITIS

Because they are a natural diuretic and have blood-cleansing properties, stinging nettles are good for relieving the painful inflammation caused by arthritis. Drink nettle tea on a daily basis or brew your own from fresh nettles.

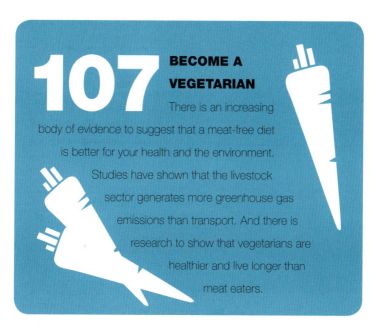

107 BECOME A VEGETARIAN

There is an increasing body of evidence to suggest that a meat-free diet is better for your health and the environment. Studies have shown that the livestock sector generates more greenhouse gas emissions than transport. And there is research to show that vegetarians are healthier and live longer than meat eaters.

108 CLEAR CONJUNCTIVITIS WITH CALENDULA

The herb calendula (*Calendula officinalis*) has antiviral and antibacterial properties, which make it ideal for treating conjunctivitis. It also has a natural cooling action, which reduces soreness. Make a compress from calendula tea and bathe the eyes.

109

RELIEVE MIGRAINES WITH GINGER

Due to its natural anti-inflammatory and pain-relieving properties, ginger may be beneficial in preventing a migraine from developing. At the first symptom, either chew on a piece of ginger root or alternatively mix a small amount of ground ginger in a glass of water and drink.

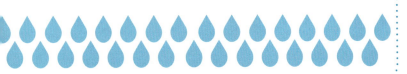

110

LET IT STAND

There is no evidence that chlorine is bad for our health but some people say it affects the taste of tap water (it is widely used to reduce bacteria). Leave a jug of tap water in the fridge for a couple of hours before drinking and this will allow the chlorine to evaporate.

111

DON'T OVERDO THE MINERALS

Despite it being marketed as the ultimate healthy drink, a recent study has shown that some mineral waters contain too much sodium and should be avoided by people with high blood pressure. Other contaminants including benzene have been found in bottled water.

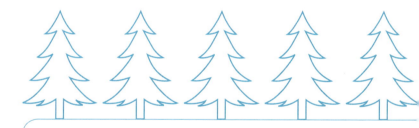

112

COOL YOUR HOME NATURALLY

Avoid the energy use and potential health hazards of air conditioning and fans and cool your home naturally. Make sure your home is well insulated, use reflective barriers such as light colour paint for the exterior to reflect heat away and use shading from blinds as well as trees and shrubs.

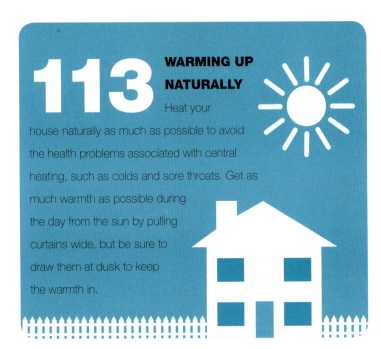

113

WARMING UP NATURALLY

Heat your house naturally as much as possible to avoid the health problems associated with central heating, such as colds and sore throats. Get as much warmth as possible during the day from the sun by pulling curtains wide, but be sure to draw them at dusk to keep the warmth in.

114

WRAP UP

Instead of flicking on the central heating as soon as the weather gets cold, which has been reported to increase your chances of developing a blocked nose and nose bleeds, put on some extra layers of clothes. Wrapping up is a healthier way of staying warmer.

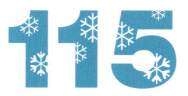

115

MAKE SURE YOU'RE INSULATED

Living in a cold, damp environment is not good for your health, and there will be times when the central heating is necessary. Make sure you're not wasting any of the energy used to heat your home by increasing the insulation in your loft.

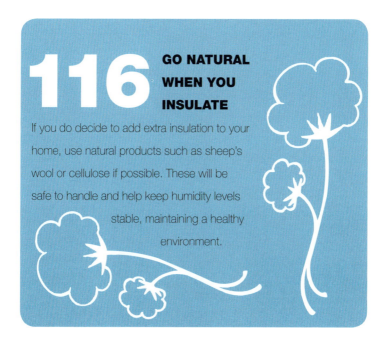

116

GO NATURAL WHEN YOU INSULATE

If you do decide to add extra insulation to your home, use natural products such as sheep's wool or cellulose if possible. These will be safe to handle and help keep humidity levels stable, maintaining a healthy environment.

117

VENTILATE YOUR HOME WELL

A cold, draughty house is not very welcoming, but it is important to ventilate your home properly as well as to draught-proof it. Inadequate ventilation in kitchens and bathrooms can cause health problems due to a potential build-up of mould.

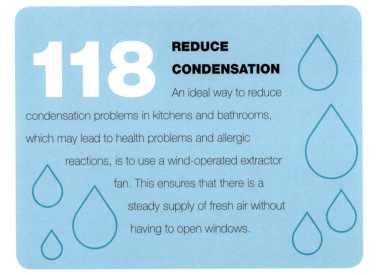

118

REDUCE CONDENSATION

An ideal way to reduce condensation problems in kitchens and bathrooms, which may lead to health problems and allergic reactions, is to use a wind-operated extractor fan. This ensures that there is a steady supply of fresh air without having to open windows.

119 GO GREEN ON YOUR ROOF

If possible, think about installing a turf roof. This will help improve the air quality around your home and provide a constant temperature, which will be good for your health and the environment. It will also help encourage biodiversity and act as a natural insulator.

120 CHOOSE CHYWANAPRASH

Chywanaprash is a traditional Indian food supplement, which is thought to help boost health during the winter months. It is made from fruit, spices, herbs and honey, and contains the amla fruit, which is a rich natural source of vitamin C and antioxidants. Often referred to as Indian gooseberry, the amla fruit contains 30 times the amount of vitamin C found in oranges, making it useful for treating throat and respiratory tract infections. Chywanaprash can be mixed with water to drink as a tea, it can be taken by the teaspoon, or can be spread on toast.

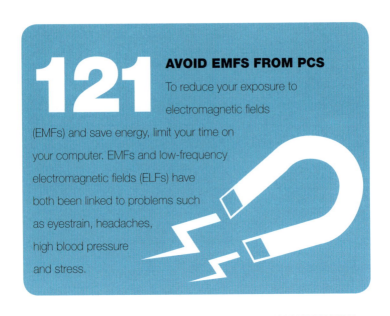

121

AVOID EMFS FROM PCS

To reduce your exposure to electromagnetic fields (EMFs) and save energy, limit your time on your computer. EMFs and low-frequency electromagnetic fields (ELFs) have both been linked to problems such as eyestrain, headaches, high blood pressure and stress.

122

UNPLUG ELECTRONIC EQUIPMENT

Although there is no proof that EMFs and ELFs are harmful, the amount of research is growing. You can reduce the levels you and your family are exposed to by switching off electrical equipment such as computers and televisions, which will also save energy.

123 BALANCING IONS

Electrical equipment such as PCs produce positive ions, which have been reported to cause atmospheric pollution and which have been linked to health problems such as hayfever and stress. To neutralize the positive ions, place some plants or a water feature near your computer.

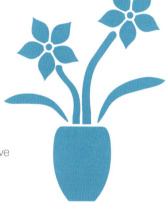

124 REDUCING STATIC

Home computers and other electrical equipment produce radiation, which has been linked to miscarriage and facial rashes. Reduce the amount of time you spend in front of your PC by switching off and going for a walk, rather than sitting at your desk with it on standby.

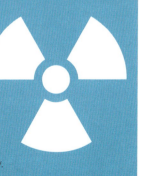

125

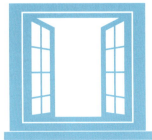

OPEN THE WINDOW

Reduce the amount of static produced by your PC by improving ventilation. Opening a window will help to prevent the build-up of static electricity. Using natural materials, such as wood, near your PC will also help the static to disperse.

126

WATCH OUT FOR RSI

Repetitive Strain Injury (RSI) is a computer-related health problem caused by working on a PC for long periods of time. Improve your health and reduce energy consumption by taking regular breaks away from your computer and stretching your arms and shoulders.

127 TAKING THE STRAIN

Prevent eyestrain from your monitor by buying one with a liquid crystal display (LCD) screen. The LCD monitors cause less strain than those with cathode ray tubes (CRT) because they are higher resolution. Plus they emit much less radiation and are slightly more energy efficient.

128 TRY NATURAL ANTIBIOTICS

There are reports of pharmaceutical antibiotics occurring in our wastewater. They have also been linked to breast cancer, Crohn's disease and childhood asthma. Avoid using them when possible by opting for natural alternatives, such as garlic, a natural antibiotic, or echinacea to build up your immmunity.

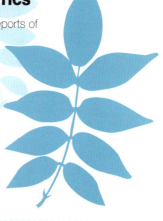

129

RELIEVE PAIN WITH ACUPUNCTURE

One of the most researched natural therapies is acupuncture, which has been found to have great success in treating everything from aches and pains to infertility. Make sure you visit a registered practitioner with a good track record.

130

TEA TREE FOR CUTS

Treat minor cuts and scratches with tea tree oil. Either dab on diluted tea tree essential oil or use a specially formulated tea tree ointment. It can also be used for insect bites, stings and blisters.

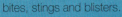

131 BRIGHTEN UP

Combat Seasonal Affective Disorder (SAD) and save energy by making the most of natural light in your home. Natural daylight is an important trigger for the production of serotonin, a brain chemical that controls mood.

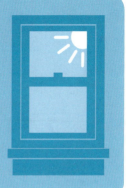

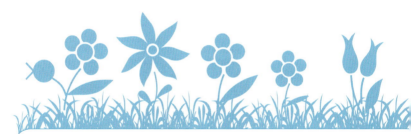

132 GET OUTSIDE

Try to spend 30 minutes a day outdoors, no matter what the weather is, and exercise regularly. This will help to lift your spirits due to the release of endorphins, boost your fitness levels and save energy on usage of household appliances at the same time.

133

USE TIGER BALM

If you have a headache try Tiger Balm before reaching for the paracetamol. This blend of Chinese herbs is a mild analgesic, which helps to promote blood flow and reduce irritation. It is also good for muscular aches and pains.

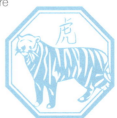

134

TEST YOUR REFLEXES

Reflexology is a natural therapy that may help a wide range of health problems without the use of pharmaceuticals. Visit a qualified practitioner first and then, if it works for you, try learning some of the pressure points yourself so you can self-treat.

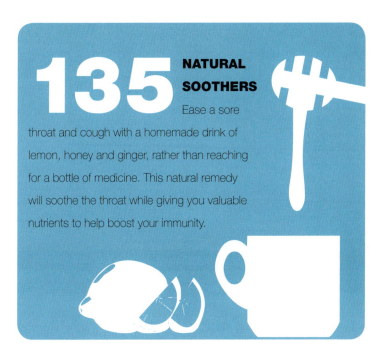

135

NATURAL SOOTHERS

Ease a sore throat and cough with a homemade drink of lemon, honey and ginger, rather than reaching for a bottle of medicine. This natural remedy will soothe the throat while giving you valuable nutrients to help boost your immunity.

136

FIGHT ACNE WITH OILS

Squeezing can make pimples worse; try treating spots with a dab of tea tree oil instead. A mixture of tea and lavender essential oils can also be dabbed directly onto blemishees a few times a day – the lavender helps to heal blemishes while the tea tree fights infection.

137 DISCOVER YOUR DOSHA

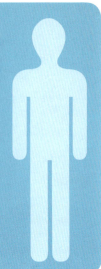

Ayurvedic medicine has been used in India for centuries. It works on the principle that we all fall into one of three 'doshas' or body types. A holistic, traditional form of medicine, Ayurvedia treats the whole body, not just the symptoms, with a combination of herbal formulations, nutrition, yoga and massage.

138 USE AROMATHERAPY

Treat minor aches and ailments with aromatherapy. This is the practice of using the therapeutic benefits of essential oils to ease symptoms such as headaches, stress and fatigue. Visit a qualified practitioner to find out which oils are best for you, and then self-administer at home.

139 BOOST YOUR IMMUNITY NATURALLY

The herb echinacea is well known for its immune-boosting properties. Research has found that it can help reduce your chances of developing a cold and will lessen the severity of symptoms if you do become ill. Take a few drops of tincture in some water on a daily basis at the start of the cold season.

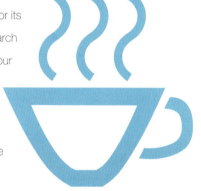

140 PUT THE FREEZE ON COLD SORES

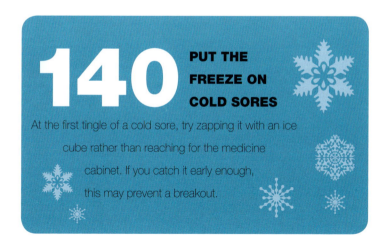

At the first tingle of a cold sore, try zapping it with an ice cube rather than reaching for the medicine cabinet. If you catch it early enough, this may prevent a breakout.

141

TREAT COLD SORES WITH TEA TREE

Both cold sores and warts can be treated with tea tree essential oil. It has powerful antiviral properties, which help dry up the blisters and eliminate warts. Mix it with an equal amount of vegetable oil to prevent irritation of the surrounding skin.

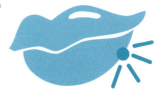

142

GET AN ALOE PLANT

The aloe vera plant is a fantastic natural cure-all. The gel can be used as an alternative to shaving foam, and it can also be applied straight to cuts and scrapes for instant relief. It has natural anti-inflammatory and skin-softening properties, which also makes it the perfect after-sun treatment.

143 NATURAL HERB HELP

Instead of using conventional pharmaceuticals, try herbalism – 80% of the world's population uses it for some aspect of primary health care. Organic herbal tinctures are free of pesticides and some are extremely effective for everyday health problems, such as feverfew for migraines.

144 USE BORAX FOR FLEAS

If you find your pet has fleas, try using borax instead of reaching for a powerful insecticide. To get rid of fleas on furnishings, sprinkle a thin later onto carpets, leave overnight and vacuum away in the morning.

145

AVOID VOCS IN LICE PRODUCTS

Conventional head lice treatments are insecticides and contain chemicals including organophosphates – a volatile organic compound (VOC). VOCs have been linked to lots of health problems including fatigue, joint and muscle pain and depression. Use a lice comb to remove lice and their eggs.

146

HERBAL HELP FOR LICE

Use shampoos made from natural plant-based ingredients, which contain essential oils such as neem to combat head lice. Try adding essential oils such as thyme – a natural insecticide – and rosemary to natural neem shampoo for an extra boost. Saturating the hair with olive oil before combing through with a lice comb is an alternative method. The oil is meant to smother the lice.

147

BEWARE OF TAKING TOO MANY MEDICINES

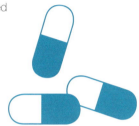

A large amount of any medicine we take is excreted in our urine. This means that there is a risk of pharmaceuticals ending up in our waterways and adversely affecting the ecosystem. To protect yourself and the environment, avoid taking more medication than you need.

148

GET A HOMEOPATHIC FIRST AID KIT

Homeopathy is a natural remedy that is based on the principle of treating like with like. Because it is safe to use on children and babies, keeping a homeopathic first aid kit in the house is a good way to look after the family without reaching for the medicine cabinet first.

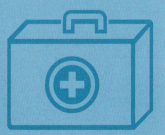

149

USE ARNICA FOR BRUISES

If you use just one homeopathic remedy, make it arnica. It is well known for it's ability to improve the healing process after injury and can be beneficial for bruising. It is the ideal remedy to administer to children after bumps to aid recovery.

150

REACH FOR THE RESCUE REMEDY

Bach flower remedies are a natural way of treating a wide range of emotional conditions, from anxiety to fear. The remedies are derived from plants and flowers and

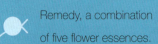

the best known is Rescue Remedy, a combination of five flower essences.

151 A TASTE OF HONEY

Eating honey is good for your health because it is high in antioxidants, which help to boost the immune system, and rich in vitamins and minerals. Bees themselves are good for the environment because they pollinate over 60 different types of crop, including fruits and vegetables.

152 EAT HONEY, AVOID HAY FEVER

There is some evidence that eating locally grown honey may desensitize you to local plant allergens, which cause hay fever. The added benefit is that buying local will reduce food miles and help support producers and the economy in your community.

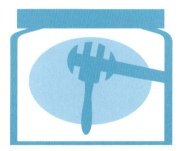

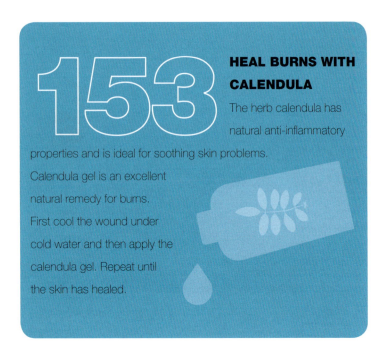

153

HEAL BURNS WITH CALENDULA

The herb calendula has natural anti-inflammatory properties and is ideal for soothing skin problems. Calendula gel is an excellent natural remedy for burns. First cool the wound under cold water and then apply the calendula gel. Repeat until the skin has healed.

154

SOOTHE SKIN WITH CHAMOMILE

The herb chamomile is known for its cleansing and cooling properties, and it is good for easing irritated skin caused by eczema or psoriasis. As a natural antihistamine and a good substitute for hydrocortisone in cases of eczema, chamomile cream will help reduce irritation and itching.

155 EASE STUFFINESS WITH EUCALYPTUS

Dilute a few drops of eucalyptus essential oil in a bowl of hot water and use as a steam inhalation to help clear nasal and sinus congestion. A few drops of eucalyptus on a handkerchief or even a pillow can aid sleep. The main ingredient of eucalyptus oil, cineole, has been studied as a treatment for sinusitis, and the oil is said to act on receptors in the nasal mucous membranes, leading to a reduction in nasal stuffiness.

156 TRY CELADRIN TO EASE ARTHRITIS PAIN

Derived from all-natural, esterified oils, Celadrin is a natural pain reliever and 'cellular lubricant' that has been found to be particularly beneficial for arthritis and joint pain caused by inflammation. It is a healthier but effective alternative to the non-steroidal anti-inflammatories that are normally prescribed, which often cause side effects such as headaches and heartburn.

157 SOOTHE SORE EYES WITH FENNEL

Eyes that are overtired or strained from working on a computer can be soothed with a solution of the herb fennel. Mix a teaspoon of fennel seeds a cup of boiling water, allow to cool, then strain. Soak a cotton wool ball in the solution and apply the compress to the eyelids for ten minutes. Fennel is also helpful for digestive ailments and relieving water retention.

158 DETOX WITH MILK THISTLE

Detoxing your body is a great way to stay healthy and rejuvenate your whole system. Before you embark on a detox programme, however, give the process a kickstart by supplementing with a tincture of the herb milk thistle, which is thought to aid detoxification by supporting the liver-cleansing process. Milk thistle has been used medicinally for over 2,000 years, most commonly for the treatment of liver and gallbladder disorders.

159

NATURAL RELIEF FOR HANGOVERS

Rather than reaching for painkillers the morning after overindulging, try getting rid of your hangover naturally first. Bananas are an excellent source of potassium, which helps to keep the body fluids balanced, so they help remedy dehydration. They also help to control blood sugar levels, which drop the day after a drinking session. Eggs are also good, as they contain cysteine, which is said to mop up the destructive chemicals that build up in the liver when it's metabolizing alcohol.

160

SPEED RECOVERY WITH VITAMIN C

Vitamin C is an excellent nutrient for speeding up recovery from a hangover. Foods naturally high in vitamin C include oranges, papaya, mango, red or orange pepper and broccoli, or you could take a vitamin C supplement instead. Avoid smoking as this will reduce levels of vitamin C in your body.

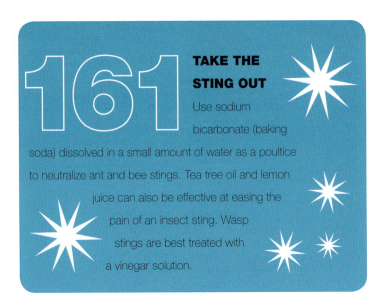

161

TAKE THE STING OUT

Use sodium bicarbonate (baking soda) dissolved in a small amount of water as a poultice to neutralize ant and bee stings. Tea tree oil and lemon juice can also be effective at easing the pain of an insect sting. Wasp stings are best treated with a vinegar solution.

162

REPEL MOSQUITOS WITH ESSENTIAL OILS

Bites from mosquitos can itch badly and become infected; avoid mosquitoes by dabbing the edges of your clothing with lavender or citronella essential oil. Another effective way to avoid mozzie bites is to eat Marmite (yeast-extract spread) – some sources say it's the lingering smell that repels them, while others say it is the folic acid in the spread.

163

TREAT CUTS WITH FRESH GARLIC

Traditionally garlic has been used to help heal cuts and wounds as it has natural antiseptic properties that boost the healing process. Rub a cut clove of garlic over the area, or place finely cut slivers onto the affected area as a poultice.

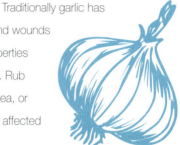

164

GET RID OF ATHLETE'S FOOT WITH TEA TREE

Tea tree oil is a natural antifungal and can be used to fight infections such as athlete's foot. Simply dab some diluted tea tree oil onto the affected area twice a day. It can also be used to prevent attacks by adding a few drops to your bath or a foot soak.

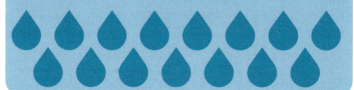

165 AVOID SICK BUILDING SYNDROME

Indoor air pollution, or Sick Building Syndrome, has been linked to all sorts of health problems such as headaches, nausea, asthma and even cancer. Try to keep your interiors as natural as possible and make sure your home is well ventilated to reduce pollution.

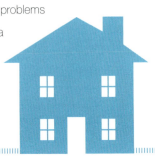

166 SAND YOUR FLOOR

A wooden floor is a green and healthy option, especially if you are sanding existing floorboards, and it is the natural alternative to synthetic carpets and vinyl. It will reduce your exposure to toxic chemicals such as volatile organic compounds (VOCs) that may be emitted by floor coverings.

167 BEWARE OF ALUMINIUM PACKAGING

Avoid buying foods packaged in aluminium or using aluminium cookware, as some reports have linked aluminium foil to low zinc levels and to premature senility and memory loss. It is estimated that the average person takes in between 3 and 10 milligrams of aluminium per day, and it can be absorbed into the body through the digestive tract, the lungs and the skin.

168 PROTECT YOURSELF WITH SOLVENT-FREE PAINT

Ecos Organic Paints are made using natural ingredients and are VOC-free. They also do a range of specialist paints to help you create a healthier home, such as their radiation-shielding wall paint and the MDF passivating primer, which is designed to absorb formaldehyde from the wood.

169

AVOID VINYL FLOORS

PVC or vinyl flooring creates environmental hazards, mainly because one of its main constituents, chlorine, can lead to the creation of dioxin – a toxin linked to cancer – when it is manufactured. Chemicals called phthalates can also leak out of PVC floors and these have been linked to asthma. A study from the *American Journal of Public Health* found that children raised in houses with PVC flooring were 89% more likely to develop bronchial obstructions.

170

WAX AWAY

If you do decide to sand your floorboards, make sure that you choose an environmentally friendly way to finish them. Waxing floorboards is the most eco-friendly option. Lots of floor varnishes contain high levels of VOCs that have been linked with asthma and other health problems.

171 KEEP YOUR WINDOWS OPEN

If you have been decorating with paint or varnish, make sure you keep your windows and doors open to reduce air pollution in your home. Conventional paints can emit possible carcinogens such as toluene and xylene, as well as hormone-disrupting chemicals. Opt for natural, ecological decorating materials, but still make sure the room is ventilated.

172 DISPOSE OF FITTED CARPETS

Wall-to-wall carpets may look comfortable but they harbour dust, which may lead to a build-up of dust mites and act as a trigger for asthma and other allergies. Replacing fitted carpets with natural flooring, such as wood, will reduce your exposure to potential allergens.

173

BEWARE OF 'GENDER BENDING' CHEMICALS IN YOUR HOME

A number of chemicals found in a huge number of household items, from paint to detergents, have become known as 'gender benders'. This is because they have been found to mimic the female hormone oestrogen. They have been linked to infertility and one group, dioxins, are known carcinogens.

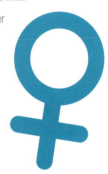

174

CHOOSE SHUTTERS INSTEAD OF CURTAINS

Although curtains are good for blocking out draughts and insulating windows, they also absorb toxins and dust. They are also likely to have been treated with flame-retardants and other chemicals to meet current fire safety regulations. If you are lucky enough to have them, wooden shutters are a better option and they are easier to clean, too.

175

AVOID TOXIC PAINTS IN YOUR HOME

Conventional paints contain solvents that give off volatile organic compounds (VOCs). These have been linked to a number of health problems including damage to the respiratory system and headaches. Always choose plant-based decorating paint made using natural ingredients.

176

BEWARE OF PLASTIC

Our homes contain plastic in a huge variety of different forms – furniture construction, paint, food containers and cleaning products. Not only is it a by-product of the energy-intensive petroleum industry, it has also been linked to health problems due to the chemicals it contains, such as Bisphenol A.

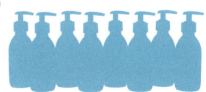

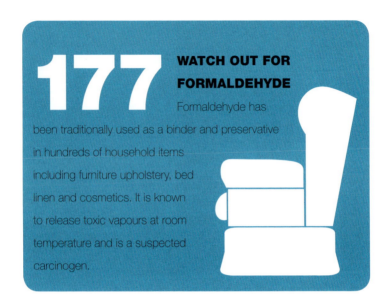

177

WATCH OUT FOR FORMALDEHYDE

Formaldehyde has been traditionally used as a binder and preservative in hundreds of household items including furniture upholstery, bed linen and cosmetics. It is known to release toxic vapours at room temperature and is a suspected carcinogen.

178

GROW YOUR OWN

Try growing your own herbs to use medicinally at home. A herb garden or even a couple of plant pots on a windowsill will enable you to brew up fresh herbal teas at home. Try feverfew for headaches and peppermint to aid digestion. There are many herbalism guides available for growing, harvesting and storing medicinal plants, as well as making remedies for home use.

179

LOOK OUT FOR LEAD

Lead can cause poisoning and is extremely energy-intensive to produce. Avoid any exposure by taking extra care when stripping old paint, which may contain high levels of lead. Use a mask to protect your nose and mouth and make sure the room is well ventilated.

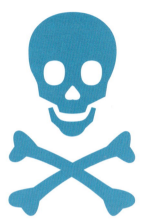

180

GET A DEHUMIDIFIER

Dehumidifiers work by removing the moisture in the air, which can cause mould, which in turn exacerbates allergies and helps to increase the dust mites in your home. A wide range of dehumidifiers are available suitable for every space from a box room to a three-bedroom house.

181

AVOID EASY-CARE CLOTHES

A reduction in the amount of ironing you need to do may sound like a good idea, but avoid fabrics that are labelled non-iron as they may have been treated with formaldehyde and could cause an allergic reaction.

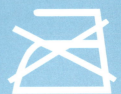

182

GO FOR ORGANIC UNDERWEAR

Conventional cotton production uses a vast amount of pesticides and there is always the chance that pesticide residue on the clothing may cause skin irritations and allergic reactions. Choose organic cotton for the sake of the environment and your skin.

183 LOOK FOR 'GREEN' FABRICS

Some of the most innovative designers today are working with 'green' fabrics such as recycled fleece and hemp, which is a fantastically sustainable fabric. Wearing clothing made from eco-friendly fabrics will reduce your exposure to pesticide residues and save energy.

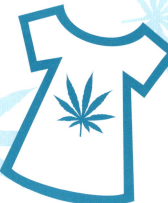

184 DON'T DRY CLEAN

Try not to choose clothes that require dry cleaning. The chemicals used in dry cleaning have been linked to health problems including dizziness, headaches and fatigue and one of them, tetrachlorethylene, is a suspected carcinogen.

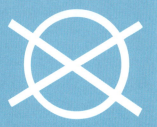

185

TRY A MAGNETIC COLLAR FOR YOUR PET

A magnetic collar can be used on cats and dogs to help improve their general well being and reduce aches and pains. They are thought to work by putting a charge in the bloodstream encouraging the blood to accept more oxygen.

186

USE GARLIC TO BANISH FLEAS

Try mincing fresh garlic into your dog's food several times a week as a natural flea repellent. Garlic has the added benefit of being an immune booster and so may help prevent other illnesses, as well as protecting against fleas and ticks.

187

REDUCE YOUR IRONING AND VACUUMING

A surprising number of cases of repetitive strain injury (RSI) are caused not by computers but by vacuuming and ironing. If there was ever a case for cutting back on two of the most tedious household chores, this is it – and you have the added bonus of saving energy, thereby cutting your carbon footprint.

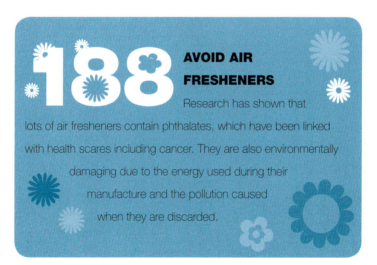

188

AVOID AIR FRESHENERS

Research has shown that lots of air fresheners contain phthalates, which have been linked with health scares including cancer. They are also environmentally damaging due to the energy used during their manufacture and the pollution caused when they are discarded.

189

OPEN UP FOR FRESH AIR

Instead of using plug-in and other synthetic air fresheners, try opening the window! Alternatively, use natural air fresheners such as cut lemon and bowls of bicarbonate of soda (baking soda), both of which will absorb whiffs without any toxic emissions.

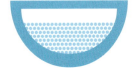

190

ESSENTIALLY YOURS

Burning essential oils and lighting scented candles are a good way to fragrance your home. Just make sure that the essential oils are organic if possible and that the candles are vegetable-oil based – paraffin candles have a much greater environmental impact and have been found to emit trace amounts of toxins.

191 MAKE YOUR OWN MOTHBALLS

Chemicals in mothballs have been found to be toxic and some are suspected carcinogens. Make your own instead, using dried herbs such as rosemary and lavender and a few drops of essential oil, all wrapped up in a piece of muslin.

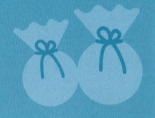

192 TRY SCENT THERAPY

Based on aromatherapy principles, these are mood-balancing patches you wear on your wrist. All-natural and easy to use, you simply bring the patch to your nose and breathe deeply three or four times. Patches are available for stress, curbing nicotine cravings, dieting and more.

193 CHOOSE FRAGRANCE-FREE PRODUCTS

Phthalates have been linked with a number of health problems including infertility and liver damage. They are commonly used in a wide range of beauty and bodycare products and are best avoided. To avoid them choose 'fragrance-free' rather than 'unscented' products, which often means that one scent has been used to mask another.

194 TAKE UP YOGA

Yoga is the eco-friendly way to unwind, tone muscles and increase flexibility. It is better than going to the gym in terms of emissions and it is fantastic for your health. Studies have shown that people who practise yoga regularly are less stressed, too.

195 GET AN OIL BURNER

Burning essential oils can improve your health and wellbeing. Use organic clove oil for mild depression and rosemary for relaxation. Peppermint essential oil can be burnt to ease nausea and stimulate the mind.

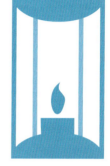

196 LAVENDER FOR RELAXATION

Add five drops of organic essential oil lavender to a bath of warm water and relax for 20 minutes. Lavender promotes relaxation and has been found to help induce a sense of calm and improve sleep.

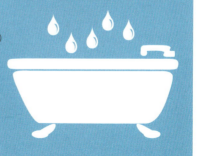

197 TREAT YOURSELF TO A MASSAGE

Massage not only provides relaxation and relief for muscle strain and fatigue, it may also provide emotional, physical and physiological benefits. It has very little impact on the environment – especially when done in candlelight – and has been found to be extremely beneficial for overall health and wellbeing.

198 CHEMICAL-FREE MASSAGE

Wooden massage tools are another way to de-stress naturally without the addition of lots of manufactured lotions and potions. Massage has been found to reduce anxiety and stress as well as boost circulation.

199 HERBAL HELP

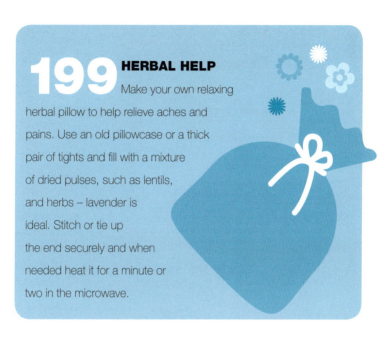

Make your own relaxing herbal pillow to help relieve aches and pains. Use an old pillowcase or a thick pair of tights and fill with a mixture of dried pulses, such as lentils, and herbs – lavender is ideal. Stitch or tie up the end securely and when needed heat it for a minute or two in the microwave.

200 UNWIND NATURALLY

For a relaxing bath, make your own bath milk. You will be able to have a long soak without worrying about exposing yourself to unnecessary chemicals, which may actually irritate and dry out the skin. Mix 2 cups of powdered milk with ½ cup of finely ground oats, and add straight to the bath for a gentle, soothing exfoliation.

201 SWAP BUBBLES FOR SALTS

Bath salts are natural and have restorative properties to relieve stress and muscle aches. They are a much greener alternative to bubble baths. Dead Sea salts have been found to help both eczema and psoriasis, and ease sore and broken skin.

202 USE OLIVE OIL ON CRADLE CAP

If your baby has cradle cap, rub some olive oil with a couple of drops of tea tree oil added onto their scalp and leave it overnight. In the morning the loose flakes can be gently brushed away with a soft baby brush. Repeat regularly until the scalp is clear.

203 BOOST FERTILITY WITH FLOWER ESSENCES

Avoid medical procedures such as IVF and boost your fertility naturally with flower remedies. The Australian bush flower remedy, she oak (*Casuarina glauca*), is thought to be especially beneficial for fertility. The plant produces fruit the same size and shape as human ovaries and has been traditionally used to boost fertility.

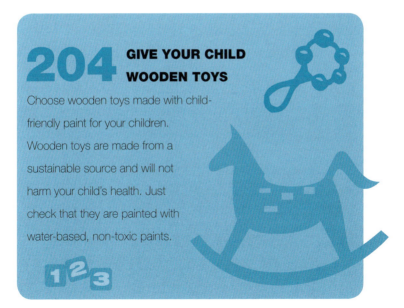

204 GIVE YOUR CHILD WOODEN TOYS

Choose wooden toys made with child-friendly paint for your children. Wooden toys are made from a sustainable source and will not harm your child's health. Just check that they are painted with water-based, non-toxic paints.

205 USE A TOOTHPASTE-FREE BRUSH

Because flouride poses health risks, especially for bone health, avoid using toothpaste altogether with an ionic eco toothbrush. These work by releasing ions, which then blend with saliva to attract positive ions from the acid in the dental plaque. The acid is neutralized, the plaque is disintegrated and there is no need for any toothpaste.

206 RINSE WITH SEA SALT

Avoid using conventional mouthwashes, which contain harsh ingredients such as alcohol and have been linked with an increase in throat and mouth cancers. Make your own rinse instead using a teaspoon of sea salt dissolved in a cup of warm water. Sea salt has natural antiseptic properties to protect the gums.

207 PICK A PLANT-BASED TOOTHPASTE

Toothpaste is a daily essential so it makes sense to choose the healthiest, greenest option to reduce exposure to chemicals. Choose a paste made from natural ingredients to avoid exposure to artificial colourings and flavourings as well as unnecessary chemicals such as triclosan.

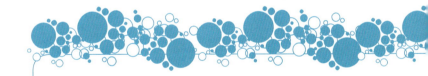

208 TAKE MORE CARE BRUSHING

Rather than relying on lots of foaming toothpaste to get your teeth clean, it would be better to ensure that you are brushing your teeth thoroughly. It is the brushing action rather than the toothpaste that gets your teeth clean, so make sure your brushing action is up to scratch.

209

USE A HERBAL MOUTHWASH

Conventional mouthwashes may contain harsh ingredients and some have even been linked with an increased risk of throat and mouth cancers. Use a natural, herbal mouthwash instead, or make your own using a few drops of sage or peppermint oil added to water.

210

USE A TONGUE SCRAPER

Rather than relying on harsh mouthwashes to maintain fresh breath, try using a tongue scraper. The bacteria that causes bad breath is often found at the back of the tongue. Regular scraping can reduce bad breath and help prevent the build-up of plaque.

211

DON'T FORGET TO FLOSS

Flossing has been shown to be very effective for good oral health, but many conventional flosses contain colourings and flavourings as well as harsh antiseptic ingredients. Look out for flosses coated in beeswax ,or vegetable waxes for vegans, rather than ingredients derived from petrochemicals. Some consist of nylon whereas others are based on pure silk strands (which may involve chemical sterilization), Teflon or other manmade fibres.

212

USE A WOODEN TOOTHBRUSH

A wooden toothbrush is kinder for the environment because it is made from a sustainable material and no plastics are involved in its manufacture. It is also easier to dispose of – you can compost or burn it in a wood burning stove. Natural bristles are also gentle on the gums, making them suitable for even very young children.

213

USE CLOVES FOR TOOTHACHE

Try using oil of cloves to relieve toothache. Dab some of the oil onto the affected area and it should numb and reduce pain, as well as helping the healing process. This may enable you to avoid taking painkillers until you have chance to visit a dentist.

214

PREVENT GUM DISEASE WITH SAGE

Regular rinsing with a solution of sage and sea salt may help protect against gum disease. Both sage and sea salt have mild antiseptic properties and have been found to reduce inflammation and promote healing. The tannins in sage are thought to help kill the bacteria that cause gingivitis.

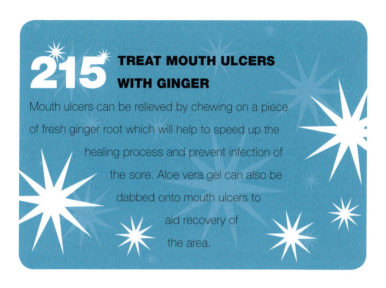

215 TREAT MOUTH ULCERS WITH GINGER

Mouth ulcers can be relieved by chewing on a piece of fresh ginger root which will help to speed up the healing process and prevent infection of the sore. Aloe vera gel can also be dabbed onto mouth ulcers to aid recovery of the area.

216 BEAT ULCERS WITH SEA SALT

Sea salt is a mild antiseptic that stimulates saliva flow and promotes self-cleaning. It also has natural healing properties, which make it good for relieving mouth ulcers. Simply gargle with a solution of sea salt in water several times a day until the ulcers have healed.

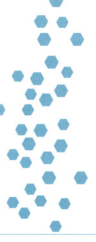

217 SUNSHINE FOR PSORIASIS

Sunshine is a natural healer for skin conditions such as psoriasis. Moderate exposure to the sun can help to heal the scaly patches that afflict sufferers, but be very careful not to burn the skin. Always avoid the sun in the middle of the day.

218 LEAVE NO TRACE

Avoid exposure to the chemical residue left on clothing by conventional detergents. This has been linked to health problems, including skin irritations and allergies. Some chemicals found in detergents are unnecessary because they don't increase the washing or hygiene effects.

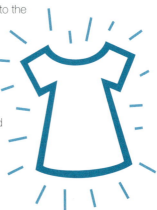

219

ALOE EASES SUNBURN

Take away the sting of sunburn with aloe vera gel. Use the purest, organic gel you can find, which will relieve pain and act as a disinfectant to protect against possible infection. Lavender oil diluted in water can also be used to clean sunburnt areas and help healing.

220

SCREEN SUN WITH EDELWEISS

The alpine plant edelweiss (*Leontopodium alpinum*) has its own built-in UV light-absorbing substance. Look out for plant-based sun lotions containing edelweiss extract for natural protection in the sun.

221

RELAX WITH REIKI

Reiki is a healing therapy that originates from Japan and involves a form of touch therapy to stimulate the life force, or *chi*. It has been found to boost relaxation and reduce stress, headaches, insomnia and improve general wellbeing.

222

WARM UP NATURALLY

Heat your house naturally to avoid the health problems associated with central heating such as colds and sore throats. Get as much warmth as possible from the sun during the day by pulling curtains wide open, but be sure to draw them at dusk to keep the warmth in.

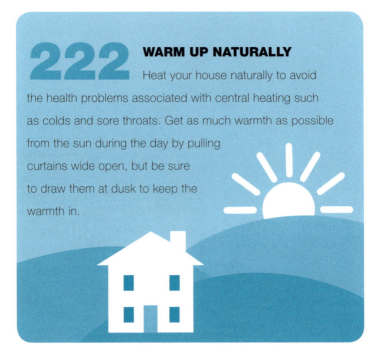

223

EAT STATIC

If you have to use a tumble dryer, avoid static on clothing by taking it out before it is 100% dry. Or use a couple of dryer balls in the dryer. These work by lifting and separating the laundry to speed up the drying time and soften clothes. This will prevent clothes from being clingy without the use of chemical-laden dryer sheets.

224

USE A NATURAL STAIN REMOVER

Reduce unnecessary exposure to the chemicals in conventional stain removers, which have been linked to a number of health problems ranging from skin irritations to cancer. Mix up your own natural stain removers using common kitchen items such as lemon juice and salt instead.

225 GET SOME SLEEP

Making sure you get enough sleep is a good way to stay healthy and boost your immune system. Lack of sleep puts extra pressure on your body and makes you susceptible to viruses. Try a cup of chamomile or valerian tea at bedtime if you have trouble sleeping. Cinnamon sprinkled onto hot milk is another good natural sleep aid.

226 COMBAT INSOMNIA WITH CHAMOMILE

If you suffer from insomnia, avoid taking sleeping pills, which have a range of side-effects. Try natural alternatives such as chamomile tea,

 which has been traditionally used to improve sleep. Put some chamomile tea bags in the bath for a sleep-inducing soak.

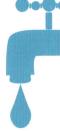

227

SLEEP EASY

If your mattress is reaching the end of it's life, why not replace it with a natural mattress? Natural, organic mattresses are free from chemicals and, as we spend roughly a third of our lives in bed, will significantly reduce your exposure to potentially toxic substances that are routinely used to treat mattresses such as fire retardants.

228

VACUUM YOUR MATTRESS

Mattresses are home to some pretty unpleasant things – including sweat from our bodies and dust mites. It is estimated that mattresses contain anything from 100,000 to 10 million dust mites, depending on their age and use. Try to air your bed as often as possible and vacuum it regularly.

229

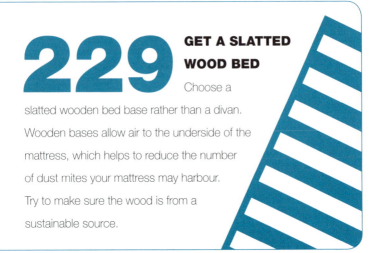

GET A SLATTED WOOD BED

Choose a slatted wooden bed base rather than a divan. Wooden bases allow air to the underside of the mattress, which helps to reduce the number of dust mites your mattress may harbour. Try to make sure the wood is from a sustainable source.

230

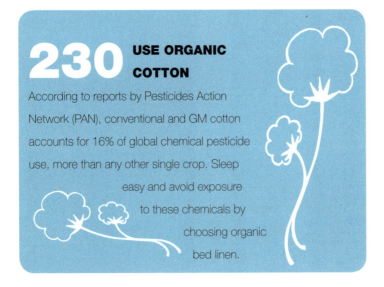

USE ORGANIC COTTON

According to reports by Pesticides Action Network (PAN), conventional and GM cotton accounts for 16% of global chemical pesticide use, more than any other single crop. Sleep easy and avoid exposure to these chemicals by choosing organic bed linen.

231 WARMING UP

Warm your bed up with a hot water bottle rather than an electric blanket. Electric blankets use unnecessary energy and have been linked with health problems. The blanket can also be a fire hazard if it develops a fault.

232 GET A HAT

The most natural and healthiest form of sun protection is to cover up. Avoid exposure to the sun, particularly during the hottest part of the day. Wear a hat, which gives good coverage to your face and neck to prevent damage to the delicate skin from the sun's rays.

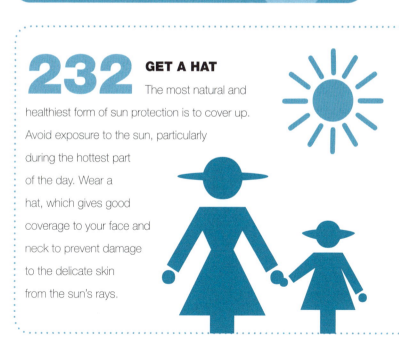

233

GET A BAMBOO COVER-UP

Make sure your children have the best sun protection by slipping on a bamboo cover-up when you are at the beach. Bamboo is a sustainable, fast-growing crop, which also provides a sun protection factor of around 50.

234

CHOOSE A NATURAL SUN BLOCK

Avoid unnecessary exposure to petrochemical-based ingredients and use a natural sun protection cream. Lots of the chemicals commonly used in sun creams are known skin irritants and some have even been found to have hormone-disrupting effects. Choose a sun cream that uses plant and mineral-based ingredients instead.

235 SEEK A GREEN DOCTOR

More GPs are getting interested in green medicine, which addresses the interplay between healthcare, the care of patients and the physician, and how sustainable development can factor into the practice of medicine. Choose one with these ideals in mind, as they may have green programmes underway.

236 CHOOSE COMPLEMENTARY MEDICINES

These are environmentally friendly if they're sourced from properly cultivated organic stock rather than harvested from wild habitats, which can disrupt the ecosystem and deplete natural resources. Make sure any treatment you get from a homeopath or naturopath is sourced in this way – not all are.

237

HELP HAY FEVER WITH EUCALYPTUS

Eucalyptus will protect you against respiratory complications and help boost your immune system during hay fever season. Like the oil, eucalyptus hydrosol is the first line of defence against respiratory problems, coughs, colds, chest infections and hay fever-type allergies. It makes a good gargle or cough syrup on its own or combined with essential oils.

238

DISPOSE DRUGS CAREFULLY

Many people flush expired medication down the toilet, thinking it's safer to do this than to dispose of it where it might be found by children or pets. Unfortunately most sewage treatment plants aren't designed to filter these drugs out, so the ingredients make their way into rivers and drinking water. Expired medication should be returned to suppliers. Pharmacies take back expired medicines, which are in turn collected by medical-waste companies that dispose of them in a responsible manner, usually by burning.

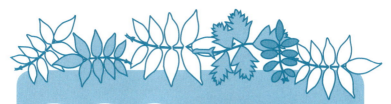

239

GO HERBAL

If you're not growing your own herbs or plant medicines, then purchasing herbal remedies or complementary medicines that are grown locally and packaged in recycled containers are better than an imported product, because they do less harm to the environment.

240

PICK PACKAGING WISELY

Packaging is another major culprit in harming the environmental. Where possible, consider eco-friendly options, including reusable packaging such as glass bottles and recyclable packaging such as glass, card and paper.

Biodegradable plastics are more environmentally friendly than the more traditional PVC plastics. Some international homeopathic brands carry a recycleable logo on their packaging, so look out for these.

241

GREEN FIRST AID

Having natural remedies on hand will help prevent you from choosing medicines that may harm the planet. Include aloe vera for wounds and burns; arnica for bruises, sprains and sore muscles; calendula for its anti-inflammatory, astringent and antiseptic qualities, and for inhibiting bleeding; camomile for an anti-inflammatory and digestion; echinacea to help fight off colds and flu; lavender oil for burns or stings; and tea tree oil for a natural antiseptic.

242

DON'T REACH FOR THE PILL

Try to modify your lifestyle or choose homeopathic remedies when you're suffering from minor illnesses rather than reaching for that headache tablet or tummy treatment. Many common ailments such as headaches, colds and indigestion are the result of poor nutritional or healthcare habits. Medicinal treatments for minor problems should be used only after all other avenues have been exhausted.

243 SIMPLE HOMEOPATHY

Keep your treatments in as pure form as possible. Homeopathic remedies are made from simple substances that, for the most part, come from the plant, animal and mineral kingdoms. Because of the method of preparation used, only small amounts of any substance are necessary to produce high-quality remedies, which means the process is unlikely to strip the earth of resources or harm animals.

244 REDUCE SNUFFLES WITH WATER

If you are feeling stuffy from a cold, place a bowl of water by the bed overnight. This will help increase the level of humidity in the room, which prevents your nasal passages from drying out and should make it easier to breathe. When you close the windows and turn the heat on in the winter, you reduce the humidity in your home, so keep air circulating to increase humidity and prevent dry skin and scratchy throats.

245 REMEDY HEADACHES

Tension headaches, caused by stress, nervous tension, eyestrain or muscular strain, can be irritating but try a natural remedy before a painkiller. Lavender and valerian are good herbal choices, or you can try immersing your feet in hot water for 15 minutes while, at the same time, applying a cold ice-water compress to your forehead, temples, back of neck, or where you feel the pain. This will increase blood flow to the feet while constricting blood vessel in the head.

246 MASSAGE AWAY HEADACHE PAIN

Place your fingers at the top of your spinal column, where your neck meets the skull. Then move your fingers out 5 cm (2 in) along the base of your skull until you find a small little indentation. Apply firm pressure with your fingers, making a small rotating motion. Breathe deeply while you massage for one to three minutes, and let yourself relax.

247

INDIGESTION AND STOMACH PAIN

Stomach discomfort is often caused by inflammation of the lining of the gut. The single best natural healing agent is aloe vera, which is available in juice form. It is rich in mucopolysaccharides, which help block pain, and it alleviates symptoms of irritable bowel syndrome (IBS).

248

CRAMPING RELIEF

If you suffer from menstrual cramps, try evening primrose oil, which is rich in gamma-linoleic acid (GLA), an anti-inflammatory prostaglandin that can counter the hormones causiong pain. Niacin (vitamin B3) is also often recommended for dilating the blood vessels and improving blood flow to the uterus.

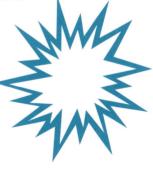

249 SPORTS INJURY HELP

One of the best anti-inflammatory painkillers for the joints and for sports injuries is bromelain, which is actually an enzyme from fresh pineapple juice. Bromelain reduces inflammation by first breaking down fibrin, a substance that would otherwise work in the body to cause local swelling. It has also been shown to be as effective as antibiotics in treating a variety of infectious and painful conditions, from bronchitis to pneumonia.

250 NATURAL STRESS RELIEF

Stress is the modern ailment that can have long-reaching effects on the body and mind, causing chronic health and mental-health conditions. To de-stress naturally, you can try meditation, massage or breathing techniques – all have a good proven track record. Take responsibility for your wellbeing, too, by making sure you are getting regular exercise, nutritional food with enough vitamin B in your diet, and a good night's sleep.